WONDERS OF CELERY:

THE AMAZING HEALING PLANT

TENDRINE WHITE

INTRODUCTION

Celery is a vegetable of the Apiaceae family. It is notable for its crunchy stalks, which individuals frequently devour as a low-calorie nibble.

In any case, in addition to the fact that celery is low in calories, however there different purposes behind adding it to the eating regimen.

It is thought to profit the stomach related tract and the cardiovascular framework, and the seeds of the plant are utilized in medication to help assuage torment.

Contents

CHAPTER ONE 1

CELERY 1

DESCRIPTION 2

CHAPTER TWO 6

USEFULNESS OF CELERY 6

LEAVES 7

SEEDS 8

CELERY SALT 9

HERBALISM 10

NUTRITION 10

MEDICAL ADVANTAGES 11

AGGRAVATION 11

PULSE 13

FORESTALLING DISEASE 14

HYPERLIPIDEMIA 15

NEUROGENESIS 17

OTHER POTENTIAL ADVANTAGES 18

CHAPTER THREE 20

NOURISHING BREAKDOWN OF   CELERY20

- DIETARY FIBER 22
- DIET 23
- CHAPTTER FOUR 26
- TIPS FOR PREPARING AND COOKING 26
- A FEW QUICK SERVING IDEAS 28
- CHAPTER FIVE 30
- DANGERS 30

CHAPTER ONE

CELERY

Celery is a vegetable of the Apiaceae family. It is notable for its crunchy stalks, which individuals frequently expend as a low-calorie nibble.

In any case, in addition to the fact that celery is low in calories, however there different explanation behind adding it to the eating regimen.

It is thought to profit the stomach related tract and the cardiovascular framework, and the seeds of the plant are utilized in medication to help calm agony.

DESCRIPTION

Celery is otherwise called Apium graveolens (A. graveolens). Different individuals from the blooming Apiaceae, or carrot, family, incorporate parsnips, parsley, and the root vegetable, celeriac. Celery leaves are pinnate to bipinnate with rhombic handouts 3–6 cm (1.2–2.4 in) long and 2–4 cm (0.79–1.57 in) expansive. The blooms are smooth white, 2–3 mm (0.079–0.118 in) in measurement, and are created in thick compound umbels. The seeds are expansive ovoid to globosely, 1.5–2 mm (0.059–0.079 in) long and wide. Current cultivars have been chosen for strong petioles, leaf stalks. A celery stalk promptly isolates into "strings" which are packs of rakish collenchyma cells outside to the vascular groups

Wild celery, Apium graveolens var. graveolens, develops to 1 m (3.3 ft) tall. It happens far and wide. The principal development is thought to have occurred in the Mediterranean locale, where the regular living spaces were salty and wet, or damp soils close to the coast where celery developed in agropyro-rumicion-plant communities.

North of the alps wild celery is discovered uniquely in the lower region zone on soils with some salt substance. It lean towards soggy or wet, supplement rich, sloppy soils. It can't be found in Austria and is progressively uncommon in Germany

Cultivar	Image	Name
Celery		*Apium graveolens* var. *graveolens*
Celeriac		*Apium graveolens* var. *rapaceum*
Leaf celery		*Apium graveolens* var. *secalinum*

CHAPTER TWO

USEFULNESS OF CELERY
Celery seed (Apium graveolens)

Celery is eaten far and wide as a vegetable. In North America the fresh petiole (leaf stalk) is utilized. In Europe the hypocotyl is utilized as a root vegetable. The leaves are firmly enhanced and are utilized less frequently, either as a seasoning in soups and stews or as a dried herb. Celery, onions, and chime peppers are the "blessed trinity" of Louisiana Creole and Cajun cooking. Celery, onions, and carrots make up the

French mirepoix, frequently utilized as a base for sauces and soups. Celery is a staple in numerous soups, for example, chicken noodle soup. Phthalides happen normally in celery.

Celery squeeze supposedly has detoxifying advantages and interest for celery spiked in 2019.

LEAVES
Celery leaves are every now and again utilized in cooking to add a gentle fiery flavor to sustenances, like, however milder than dark pepper. Celery leaves are

reasonable dried as a sprinkled on flavoring for use with prepared, fricasseed or cooked fish, meats and as a feature of a mix of crisp seasonings appropriate for use in soups and stews. They may likewise be eaten crude, blended into a plate of mixed greens or as a topping.

SEEDS
In calm nations, celery is additionally developed for its seeds. In reality little organic product, these "seeds" yield a profitable fundamental oil that is utilized in

the fragrance business. The oil contains the concoction compound apiole. Celery seeds can be utilized as enhancing or flavor, either as entire seeds or ground.

CELERY SALT
The seeds can be ground and blended with salt, to create celery salt. Celery salt can be produced using a concentrate of the roots or utilizing dried leaves. Celery salt is utilized as a flavoring, in mixed drinks (prominently to improve the kind of Bloody Mary mixed drinks),

on the Chicago-style wiener, and in Old Bay Seasoning.

HERBALISM

Celery seeds have been utilized broadly in Eastern natural customs, for example, Ayurveda.[25] Aulus Cornelius Celsus composed that celery seeds could assuage torment in around AD 30.

NUTRITION

Celery is used in weight loss diets where it provides low calorie dietary fiber bulk.

MEDICAL ADVANTAGES

Celery gives fiber and supplements.

The conceivable medical advantages of celery and its seeds include:

- bringing down aggravation
- diminishing pulse
- diminishing the danger of disease
- anticipating age-related vision misfortune

AGGRAVATION

Celery contains apigenin, an atom that is presently being concentrated for its enemy of malignant growth properties.

An examination distributed in Molecular Nutrition and Food Research explored whether this substance may help adjust or decrease harm brought about by aggravation.

The creators presume that apigenin and apigenin-rich weight control plans decreased the statement of certain incendiary proteins in mice. Along these lines, they can decrease aggravation and reestablish invulnerable equalization.

PULSE

There is no solid proof that celery seeds help to lower pulse in people, however an examination distributed in the Journal of Medicinal Food demonstrated that it had this impact on rodents.

The examination took a gander at the impact of celery seed separates on pulse in rodents with typical circulatory strain and with rodents with falsely initiated hypertension.

The creators reason that:

"Celery seed concentrates have antihypertensive properties, which gives off an impression of being inferable from the activities of its dynamic hydrophobic comprises, for example, NBP (n-butylphthalide) and can be considered as an antihypertensive specialist in interminable treatment of raised BP."

The outcomes propose that celery may effectsly affect people.

FORESTALLING DISEASE
Celery contains a flavanoid called luteolin. Specialists trust that luteolin may have against malignant growth properties.

An investigation distributed in Current Cancer Drug Targets said that "Ongoing epidemiological examinations have ascribed a malignancy aversion property to luteolin."

The creators trust this happens in light of the fact that luteolin makes disease cells progressively vulnerable to assault by synthetic compounds utilized in treatment.

HYPERLIPIDEMIA

Hyperlipidemia happens when there is an expansion in greasy particles in the blood. There are frequently no indications, however it raises the long haul danger of coronary illness and stroke.

An investigation distributed in Advances in Environmental Biology analyzed whether celery concentrate may almost certainly diminish hyperlipidemia in rodents that expended a high-fat eating routine.

Results demonstrated that the concentrate did in fact lessen the measure of LDL, or "awful," cholesterol in the blood.

In spite of the fact that this is a creature ponder, on the off chance that it is reproduced in people it could give another valid justification to devour celery.

NEUROGENESIS

Apigenin is additionally accepted to animate neurogenesis, the development and advancement of nerve cells.

Research distributed in 2009 examined the impacts of apigenin in mice. Discoveries demonstrated that, when infused or taken orally, apigenin improved learning and memory.

Further investigations are expected to affirm these discoveries in people.

OTHER POTENTIAL ADVANTAGES

Celery may likewise be valuable in treating joint agony and relieving the sensory system, however there isn't sufficient logical proof to completely bolster the cases at this stage.

Celery seeds may have therapeutic properties.

The University of Maryland Medical Center (UMM) state that celery seeds have for quite some time been utilized in prescription to treat, among others:

- joint inflammation and gout
- muscle fits
- irritation
- hypertension
- colds and influenza
- water maintenance

CHAPTER THREE

NOURISHING BREAKDOWN OF CELERY

Celery is a rich wellspring of phenolic phytonutrients that have cancer prevention agent and calming properties. These phytonutrients include: caffeic corrosive, caffeoylquinic corrosive, cinnamic corrosive, coumaric corrosive, ferulic corrosive, apigenin, luteolin, quercetin, kaempferol, lunularin, beta-sitosterol and furanocoumarins. Celery is a great wellspring of nutrient K and molybdenum. It is an awesome wellspring of folate, potassium, dietary fiber, manganese and pantothenic corrosive. Celery is likewise a decent wellspring of nutrient B2, copper, nutrient C, nutrient B6, calcium, phosphorus, magnesium and nutrient An (as carotenoids).

Celery additionally contains roughly 35 milligrams of sodium for each stalk, so salt-delicate people can appreciate celery, however should monitor this sum when observing day by day sodium admission.

Nutrients and minerals: Celery is wealthy in nutrient K, and it likewise contains folate, nutrient A, potassium, and nutrient C.

DIETARY FIBER

Celery is basically water, however it is likewise a decent wellspring of dietary fiber. One measure of cleaved celery, or 100 grams of celery, identical to around more than two medium stalks, contains 1.6 grams of fiber.

DIET

Celery can be eaten crude or cooked. Studies demonstrate that it loses almost no of its supplements when steamed.

Celery makes a solid expansion to smoothies.

In 2011, researchers distributed research that inspected the loss of absolute phenolic cancer prevention agent supplements from celery when whitened for 3 minutes, steamed for 10 minutes, and bubbled for 10 minutes.

Bubbling and whitening brought about huge cancer prevention agent misfortunes, between 38 percent and 41 percent. In the wake of steaming, be that as it may, celery held 83 percent to 99 percent of its cell reinforcements.

Celery can be eaten with cheddar, with plunges, in plates of mixed greens, or as a crunchy expansion to a nutty spread sandwich.

It additionally adds flavor to soups and risottos. Pursue the connections for certain plans suggested by dietitians:

Tomato chicken soup with carrots and celery

Braised celery

Joined with cucumber, apple, spinach, and lemon, celery makes a delectable and stimulating expansion to a smoothie.

Celery seeds can be added to vegetable dishes, soups, and serving of mixed greens dressings for flavor.

Celery's cousin, celeriac, includes in White bean and celery root gratin with bulghur outside layer.

CHAPTTER FOUR

TIPS FOR PREPARING AND COOKING

Tips for Preparing Celery

To clean celery, remove the base and leaves, at that point wash the leaves and stalks under running water. Cut the stalks into bits of wanted length. On the off chance that the outside of the celery stalk has sinewy strings, evacuate them by making a meager cut into one end of the stalk and stripping without end the filaments. Make certain to utilize the leaves—they contain the most nutrient C, calcium, and potassium—yet use them inside multi day or two as they don't store great.

Celery ought not be kept at room temperature for over a few hours. That is on the grounds that warm temperatures will energize its high water substance to vanish, making the celery have tend to shrink too rapidly. On the off chance that you have celery that has withered, sprinkle it with a little water and spot it in the cooler for a few hours to enable it to recover a portion of its freshness.

A FEW QUICK SERVING IDEAS

Add hacked celery to your preferred fish or chicken plate of mixed greens formula.

Appreciate the delightful custom of eating nutty spread on celery stalks.

Use celery leaves in plates of mixed greens.

Braise slashed celery, radicchio and onions and serve beat with pecans and your preferred delicate cheddar.

Next time you are making crisp crushed carrot juice give it a novel taste measurement by adding some celery to it.

Include celery leaves and cut celery stalks to soups, stews, meals, and Healthy Stir-Fries.

Consider the buy of celery in its non-Pascal assortments. Root celery can be filled in as a noteworthy plate vegetable all its own, and leaf celery can be substituted for parsley in practically any formula.

CHAPTER FIVE

DANGERS

Celery has a place with a little gathering of sustenances that can cause a serious hypersensitive response, and this can prompt deadly anaphylactic stun.

The individuals who are adversely affected by the celery ought to be wary and check sustenance names, as even little hints of celery can cause a response.

Celery likewise has a generally high sodium content, at 35 milligrams for each stalk. Be that as it may, this is almost no contrasted and the 1,500 milligrams daily suggested by the American Heart Association, and far not exactly the 3,400 milligrams daily devoured by generally Americans. It is as yet a low-sodium nourishment.

www.ingramcontent.com/pod-product-compliance
Lightning Source LLC
Chambersburg PA
CBHW030548220526
45463CB00007B/3034